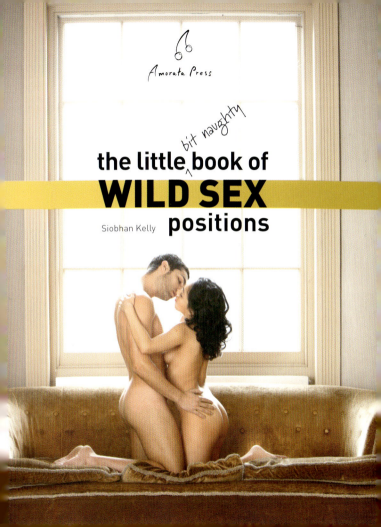

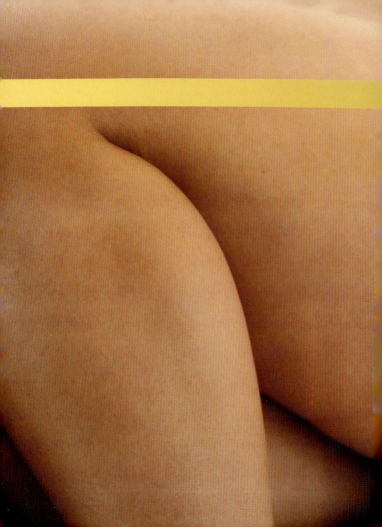

Let's go outside

Because bedrooms can get boring...

Taking your love-making on location is a great way to open your mind and body to new sex positions you wouldn't normally try on the sheets and pillows.

Here's our sizzling selection of sexperiments to liven up every room in the house...

Mild-to-wild rating: 3

THE F WORD

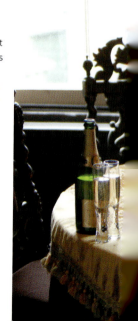

PUMP UP THE PLEASURE

Introduce a little role-play. He wears nothing but a chef's hat or apron. With a little flavoured lube and a handful of strawberries, he turns her whole body into a living fruit salad – and licks her all over to get her ready for penetration.

Combine food and sex in this delicious position. She lies back on the kitchen worktop or table with her legs raised. He stands before her and enters her, grabbing onto her legs or thighs if necessary to balance.

Thrusting and holding her up can be a lot of work for him, but this position offers deep penetration and unparalleled vaginal and clitoral stimulation. Partners can maintain eye contact throughout, and she can vary the degree of penetration by putting her feet onto his chest to make it deeper, or wrap her legs around his neck or back to increase the feeling of intimacy and involvement. If she puts her feet onto his chest, she's got a bit more leverage and is less likely to fall off. She can lower her legs towards her chest to lengthen the angle of her vagina and give longer, tighter penetration.

He says: *'Pressing the soles of her feet against my chest meant that I could really thrust hard into her.'*

She says: *'The smooth wood of the table underneath my body made me feel really alive and awoke every nerve ending in my body.'*

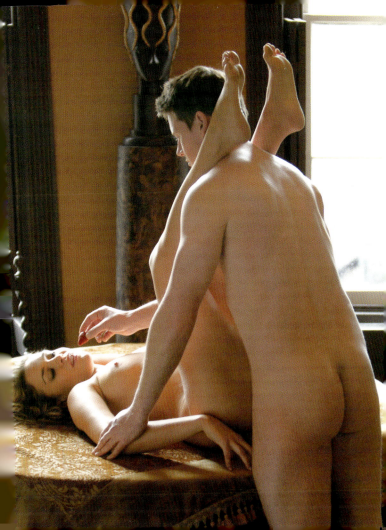

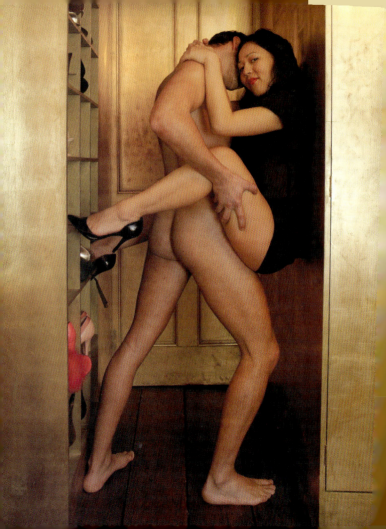

Mild-to-wild rating: 4

HARD LAY AT THE OFFICE

Ever fantasised about having sex at work? The woman-on-top position is great for quickie sex in an extremely confined space like a stationery cupboard.

He leans back against the wall or on a cabinet or shelf while she straddles him, her knees bent, bracing her feet against the wall opposite and her back against the wall behind her. Using both walls for support, she pushes away with her feet and bounces up and down on his penis. Her breasts are in optimum position for him to take into his mouth while she slides up and down his length. He can grip her rump to help support her and control the speed of her movements.

She can use her thighs to raise herself up so that only the tip of his penis is inside his vagina. Using her PC muscles to make sure he doesn't fall out, she can then gently swivel her hips from side to side before slowly sliding back down again so that the whole length of him is inside her once more.

PUMP UP THE PLEASURE

Make sure you're wearing clothes that have easy access (and make for a quick getaway if you get caught). A short skirt with panties that can be pulled aside is ideal.

He says: *'I loved that she bit down onto my shoulder to muffle her moans of ecstasy. I wore that bite mark like a badge of pride for days.'*

She says: *'There's something really urgent about doing it in a confined space. With such limited range of movement, my clit was pressed tight against his pubic bone and every sensation was so much more intense.'*

Mild-to-wild rating: 4

DOORWAY TO HEAVEN

Doorways are a much-neglected potential hotspot in the home (or hotel room, or office, or wherever you are when the urge strikes you). In this rear-entry position, you prop yourselves up on the sturdy frame, leaving all your energy to lavish upon each other. He leans back across the doorway, making a diagonal across the frame with his body. He bends his legs until his pelvis is low enough for her to straddle, and she slowly lowers herself down onto his waiting erection. Gently, she moves her body weight back while leaning on the opposite diagonal so that from the side the lovers look like the letter X. As she does this, both lovers will feel the angle of penetration become tighter and more intense.

PUMP UP THE PLEASURE

Words can be as arousing as touch. It's possible to free one hand each in this position, so why not highlight steamy passages from a favourite erotic novel and take it in turns to read aloud?

He says: *'It took a couple of minutes to get used to the tight hold she had on my dick – it felt like her whole body was bearing down on it. I was worried I might come too soon, so I reached around and played with her clitoris to speed up her climax.'*

She says: *'This is a great way to experiment with sex al fresco without actually leaving the house. We tried it in the back doorway on a hot summer's night. It's tough on the thighs, and quite strenuous, but working up a sweat only added to the intensity of the position.'*

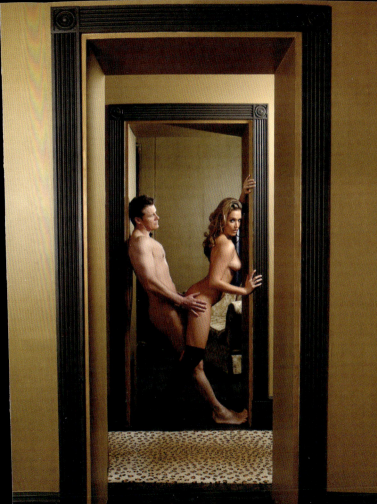

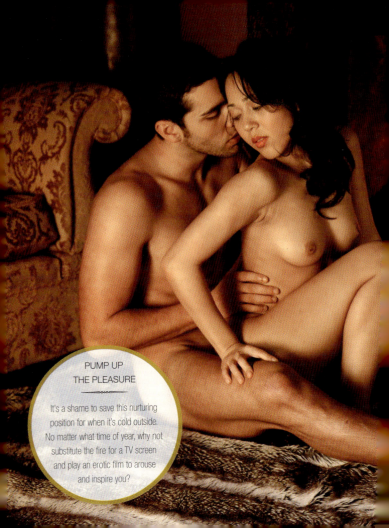

PUMP UP THE PLEASURE

It's a shame to save this nurturing position for when it's cold outside. No matter what time of year, why not substitute the fire for a TV screen and play an erotic film to arouse and inspire you?

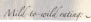

Mild-to-wild rating: 3

Winter warmer

Most of us have fantasised about making love in front of a crackling log fire. He sits with his legs outstretched in front of him. She sits in his lap, wrapping her pussy around his erect penis and then slowly leans forward. This is about gentle, incremental stimulation rather than deep thrusting, so focus on small, but stimulating circular gyrations and pulsing pussy squeezes.

She's very much in control of his pleasure here – the further forward she leans, the tighter the squeeze around his dick. He can return the treat – the back is our largest flat expanse of skin but we often neglect it as an erogenous zone. By lavishing her back, neck and shoulders with kisses, nibbles and nips, he can make her shiver – despite the fire's flames!

He says: *'Playing with her nipples so close like this was a new and exciting angle for me. I loved the weight of a breast in each hand.'*

She says: *'It didn't take long to work out that if I lean my body forward just a couple of centimetres he gets an extra squeeze that makes his whole body tingle. It's great to know I can turn him on so much with so little effort.'*

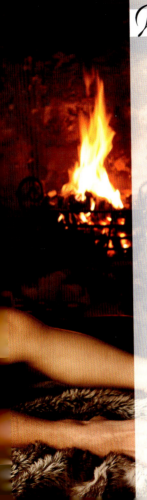

Mild-to-wild rating: 3

LOVE IN THE TUB

He lies back in the tub. Sitting astride him, she places her legs tightly against his sides, tucking her feet in under him for support. The man opens his thighs just enough for her to slip down off his lap and onto his erection. Do this slowly, allowing yourselves to feel each millimetre of penetration as it happens. Focus on the moment when the tip of his dick prises apart her pussy lips and enters for the first time.

Clutching each other's wrists, both partners lean back carefully. Keeping her knees pressed together will maintain a tight squeeze on the penis. Neither partner takes the lead in this position and, although it looks difficult, the support of the water will ease any strain. The only potential power struggle is over who gets the tap end!

He says: *'This is a great way to make love after a long and stressful day.'*

She says: *'I love the feeling of weightlessness, and I'm sure this helps me to relax and gives me a stronger orgasm.'*

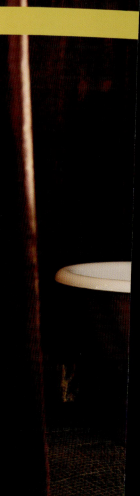

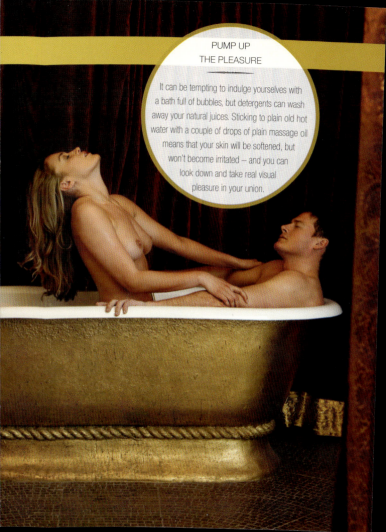

PUMP UP THE PLEASURE

It can be tempting to indulge yourselves with a bath full of bubbles, but detergents can wash away your natural juices. Sticking to plain old hot water with a couple of drops of plain massage oil means that your skin will be softened, but won't become irritated – and you can look down and take real visual pleasure in your union.

THE SOFA SUPPER

This side-by-side position is great for spontaneous but lazy sex. Lie on your sides in a simple embrace, beginning in the same foetal position. Slowly press your bodies together; his chest is close into her back. Raising her outside leg slightly, she squeezes the penis in the groove of her buttocks and with very slight movements of her pelvis she makes him hard between them. Arching her back exposes her genitals even more so that the man can rub the tip of his penis against her vulva, until she is wet and begging to take him inside her.

PUMP UP THE PLEASURE

Crack open the champagne and pass it to and from each other in a flute. One glass of sparkling wine will lower your inhibitions and up your testosterone, making for hot, horny sex. He can also drizzle the golden liquid over her breasts and belly during sex. The tiny fizzing bubbles will stimulate her skin.

Mild-to-wild rating: 3

He says: *'We often make love in this position late at night when we're chilling in front of a horny film. We can both see the screen at the same time. Sometimes we do it with the sound turned down and listen to our own moans instead.'*

She says: *'I like to stimulate my own clitoris here, holding it between my thumb and forefinger and feeling it swell as he rocks inside me. I flick it to bring myself to orgasm at just the right moment.'*

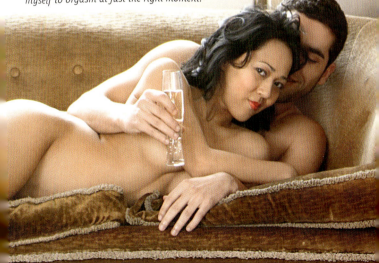

Power, pain

Bondage, domination and submission, master and mistress, slave and servant – the very words are enough to send a shiver down the spine. There can be something wonderfully liberating about surrendering to your lover's commands, and the power of watching them do your bidding can trigger intense orgasms. The positions on the following pages are designed to inject maximum psychological tension as well as physical pleasure into your power play. Whether you're in the mood to submit or dominate, to give or receive, there's a position here for you.

and pleasure

Play by the rules:
- Safety and security underpin even the most extreme power play positions.
- Don't attempt them when you're drunk or on drugs, or with someone you've just met. These positions are extreme and risky, and you need trust and good judgement.
- The intense fantasy of fetish means that sometimes you can whimper 'no' when you mean 'yes'. Have a code word with no sexual connotations that **really** means 'stop'.

MALE-DOMINANT POSITIONS

Her Master's Voice

Mild-to-wild rating: 4

She stands facing a wall, wearing heels or standing on a box or step to raise her pelvis in line with his. She presses the front surface of her body into the wall, and he bends his legs and enters her from behind, putting his whole body weight behind her so that her body is pressed flat against the wall. This position offers deep penetration for him and excellent G-spot stimulation for her. He can whisper in her ear what a bad girl she's been, and list all the ways he intends to punish her.

> **PUMP UP THE PLEASURE**
>
> To add to her feelings of complete surrender, and to amplify his sexy suggestions, he blindfolds her and guides her body into position himself.

He says: *'The master-and-slave fantasy is really horny but saying the words doesn't always come easily and we can get a bit giggly when we're face to face. When there is no eye contact, it's much easier to indulge the fantasy that I'm a stranger forcing her to have an orgasm against her will.'*

She says: *'I like to do this wearing a really high pair of heels that I got in a fetish shop in London. I can't really walk in them, but they bring my hips up to the right height for his dick and make me feel even more vulnerable because I know that I couldn't run away even if I wanted to – which I don't!'*

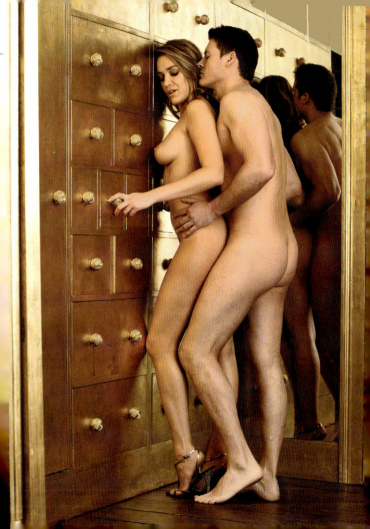

Mild-to-wild rating: 4

THE STOCKING FILLER

This tied-up tease is a great position for couples who are new to bondage as the restraints used are light and simple and the position is not physically challenging.

She lies back on the bed, spread-eagling her body so that her arms and legs are as far apart as they can go. Using a couple of pairs of her stockings, he ties her wrists and ankles to the bedposts. He allows her a little room to wriggle, and ensures that her blood can still circulate, but is firm enough so that she can't move until he unties her. He lies over her, supporting his weight on his elbows, enters her and thrusts. It's powerfully erotic, with the woman at her most open and vulnerable, and the man able to exercise his full sexual power. He controls most of the thrusting, and there's very little effort involved for her. Kissing and talking is possible throughout, as is all-important eye contact and close body contact.

He says: *'Because her legs are spread so wide, I get to see myself pumping in and out of her, which makes my erection even harder.'*

She says: *'I love the feeling of being laid out for him to explore and conquer. I've discovered all sorts of new erotic hidden places in this position, like the skin on the inside of my arms and inner thighs.'*

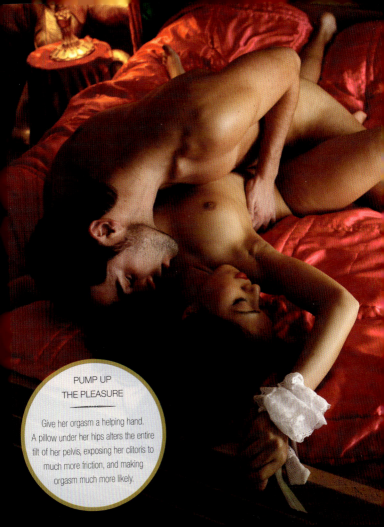

PUMP UP THE PLEASURE

Give her orgasm a helping hand. A pillow under her hips alters the entire tilt of her pelvis, exposing her clitoris to much more friction, and making orgasm much more likely.

Mild-to-wild rating: 4

ANKLE CLASP

Her hot body is on full display in this position, and she's helpless to do anything but lie back and bask in his desire and adoration.

She lies on her back, and he kneels and enters her, holding a firm grip on her ankles and spreading her legs as wide as they will go. You'll want to experiment with the most pleasing width and the pace of thrusting. Penetration will be deep and the pressure of his pelvic bone on her clitoris adds delicious friction to the mix.

He says: *'That moment when I prise her legs apart and watch her vagina open up like a flower in front of me is the biggest turn-on I can describe. Sometimes I pull out and just gaze at it. I like to leave it just long enough so that she's begging to have me inside her again.'*

She says: *'He knows just how far to push me when he stretches my legs apart. He'll hold them as far as they can go, and then he'll push them just a millimetre more with each thrust. That tiny pain in my leg muscles adds a new dimension to the pleasure in my pussy.'*

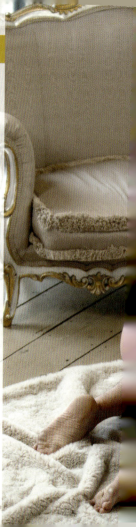

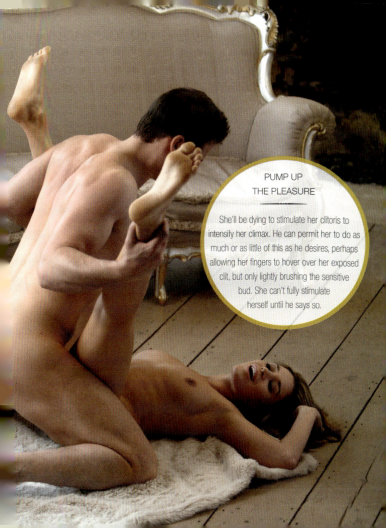

PUMP UP THE PLEASURE

She'll be dying to stimulate her clitoris to intensify her climax. He can permit her to do as much or as little of this as he desires, perhaps allowing her fingers to hover over her exposed clit, but only lightly brushing the sensitive bud. She can't fully stimulate herself until he says so.

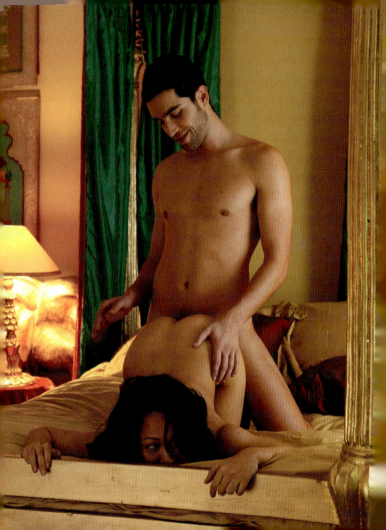

Mild-to-wild rating: 3

THE ROSY CHEEK

One of the most popular bondage role-play scenarios is the naughty student and the strict teacher who needs to instil some discipline into his charge.

She kneels on all fours, ass raised slightly in the air, her arms spread before her on the bed in a gesture of submissiveness. He kneels behind her, his knees apart, and penetrates her. He can lightly slap her bottom, watching it turn a rosy pink. There's not much scope for thrusting but this position will bring the blood flowing to her genitals and she can use that extra sensation to clench her PC muscles and give him a squeeze to climax. It's also great for G-spot stimulation.

PUMP UP THE PLEASURE

Everyone likes to give and receive different degrees of spanking. Begin with a light slap with her hand; if that turns you both on, you might want to invest in a special paddle from a sex shop. Whether you're spanking a man or a woman, it's important to slap the juicy flesh of the bottom, not the back, as that's where the vulnerable vital organs live.

He says: *'I love the moans and groans that I get from her in this position, and I love to feel the heat rush to her skin.'*

She says: *'I love the way that my tits press against the bed in this position. Sometimes, when he's not looking, I sneak one hand between my legs and caress myself, or give my breasts little pinches.'*

FEMALE-DOMINANT POSITIONS

Mild-to-wild rating: 5

ROLE REVERSAL

We're used to sex positions where the man carries the woman, but have you ever thought of reversing those roles? After all, a good mistress knows she is a strong, capable woman who understands that it's important to protect as well as punish her slave. Unless she's an Olympic weightlifter going out with a champion jockey, she will need to support him on some kind of surface that can bear his weight. The kitchen worktop, a dressing table or office desk is ideally placed to be at her hip height.

He sits on the edge; she stands opposite him and parts her legs, allowing him to penetrate her. He stabilises himself by grasping her buttocks and gently the mistress and her slave rock to orgasm.

PUMP UP THE PLEASURE

Her breasts are at his eye level in this primal position. She can enhance them by letting them spill out of a tight, lace-up corset.

He says: *'This position is really nurturing and we often use it after really dirty sex in another position, just to finish off. There's something really tender about it and after really kinky abusive sex sometimes you just want something a bit cuddlier.'*

She says: *'I order him to lower his head and suck my breasts in this position. He's only too keen to obey.'*

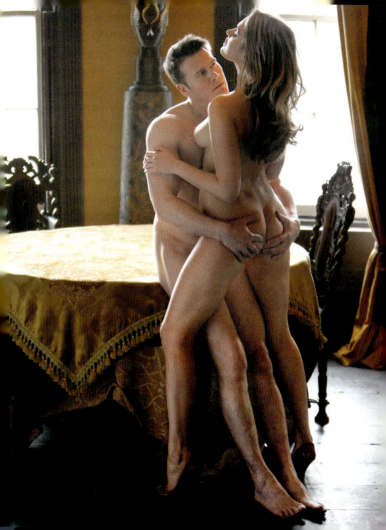

Mild-to-wild rating: 4

Heel, Boy!

This female-superior position is a treat for the man who loves sexy feet and the dominatrix who wants to show off her pedicure and/or shoe collection.

He lies on his back, knees bent, in a semi-supine position. His mistress talks dirty or masturbates him until his dick is hard and then straddles him, lowering her pussy onto his erection. She then slowly moves her legs around until they are extended in front of her, with her feet in his face. She uses her hands on his knees to stabilise herself and begins to squeeze and rock on top of his penis. She can then use her feet to tease and taunt him, whether that involves inserting a toe into his mouth, or lightly applying pressure with the sharp stab of a stiletto.

He says: *'It's my favourite view in the world. I'm getting hard now just thinking about it.'*

She says: *'Until you have your toes sucked, you have no idea how powerfully erotic it feels.'*

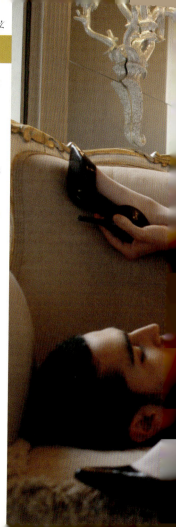

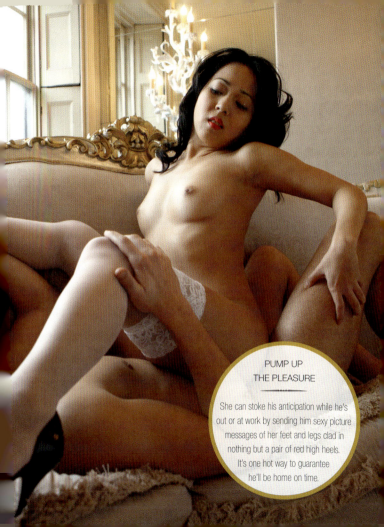

Mild-to-wild rating: 4

Bad Cop

This woman-on-top position allows him to gaze up at her in rapt adoration. Add the thrill of him being restrained, and fireworks are guaranteed.

He lies on his back and she uses handcuffs, bondage tape or even an old tie to secure his arms to the bedpost. As she restrains him, she talks to him, reminding him that he can't get away. She straddles him and gently slides herself down onto his erection and uses her thighs to move up and down. Unless she has strong thighs, this position can get tiring quickly, but she can move about and even drop down into female missionary. He may find it more comfortable if his head is propped up on pillows. She may choose to withhold this comfort, depending on how generous she's feeling and how obedient he is being.

He says: *'The only bit of your body you can really move is your hips, so that's what I kept doing – bucking them up and digging my dick as deep into her as I could. She was trying to be a strict dominatrix but she couldn't hide the pleasure every time I pushed a little deeper into her.'*

She says: *'Usually when I'm playing the mistress, I tell him to pinch my tits or play with my clit. Because his hands were tied, I had to do this myself … and that was sexy.'*

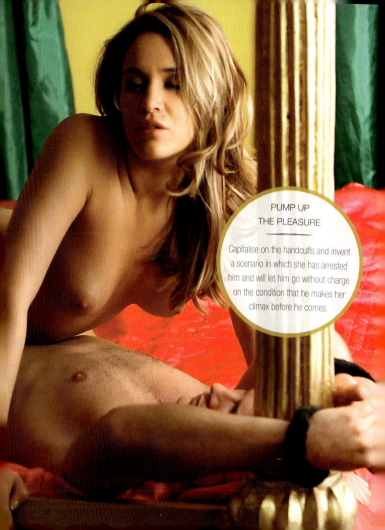

PUMP UP THE PLEASURE

Capitalise on the handcuffs and invent a scenario in which she has arrested him and will let him go without charge on the condition that he makes her climax before he comes.

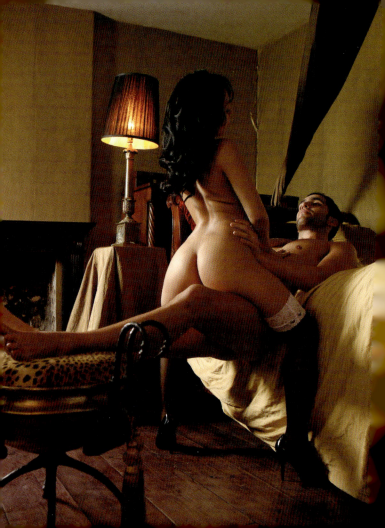

Mild-to-wild rating: 5

THE SUSPENSION BRIDGE

He lies with his back and shoulders on the bed and his feet on another surface, like a dressing table or sturdy chair, so that his body is making a kind of bridge between the two pieces of furniture. The dominatrix stands at the edge of the bed between his legs, and grabs his hips and slowly raises his pelvis until his hard-on is exactly where she wants it to be – ready to penetrate her. She can bend her legs and use her arms to rock him to orgasm. This is a great position for a strong, fit woman to revel in the power of her body, but avoid it if he's got a weak back, or if your furniture is likely to slide out from underneath him.

PUMP UP THE PLEASURE

Scatter scratchy sequins on the floor below him and tell him that it's a bed of nails. Fear of falling will add a delicious tension to the proceedings as he struggles to keep the 'bridge' in the air.

He says: 'There's a real element of trust involved in this one as I mustn't drop her, but if she puts too much of her weight on me I'd be forced to the floor. The words she said really made this one come alive, telling me she could make me fall any minute and making me promise undying allegiance to her in return for my safety.'

She says: 'His legs are supporting most of his body weight so it's not as tiring as it looks. A lot of BDSM positions are about psychology so it's nice to have one where I'm so physically dominant.'

Joy of toys

There's more to sex toys than solo masturbation, and there's more to sex positions than penis meets vagina. These positions incorporate the most popular sex toys and are great for maximum pleasure with minimum time and effort from you. They all make for delicious foreplay and can be enjoyed as a main event in themselves.

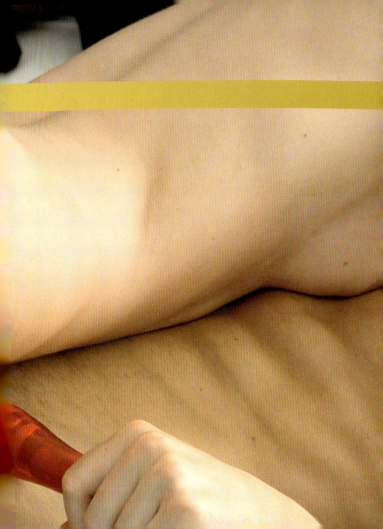

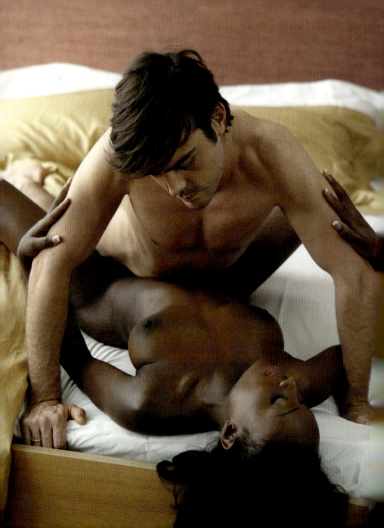

Mild-to-wild rating: 3

ADDICTED TO BUZZ

This high-tech twist on sex in the missionary position, where she lies back on the bed and he lies on top and penetrates, couldn't be simpler.

There are a lot of reasons why this plain old man-on-top position is the most popular love-making pose throughout the world – it's easy, intimate and nurturing. But it also comes with a bit of a design fault in that he controls the depth and pace of the thrusting and can reach his climax within a few minutes, while she can find it challenging to receive the clitoral stimulation she needs to reach orgasm. So take all the fuss out of it by slipping on a vibrating cock ring. These are little toys with a tiny in-built vibe that he slips over his cock and balls before entering her. The ring traps the blood in his erection, making it feel harder and last longer, and the little vibrating tip delivers a fast, furious stimulation to her clitoris that could have her climaxing in as little as 20 seconds.

PUMP UP THE PLEASURE

If you don't have a vibrating cock ring then wedging a miniature vibrator between your pubic bones creates a similar sensation.

He says: *'I am, of course, dedicated to my partner's pleasure but I have to say that it's great to let the toy do all the work. If you're really horny, but really lazy, this is ideal.'*

She says: *'The first time we tried this I came so quickly that he had barely had time to get started. Now I know that an orgasm is pretty much guaranteed, I can relax into the penetration and enjoy that as well as the clit stim.'*

Mild-to-wild rating: 4

VIBEALICIOUS

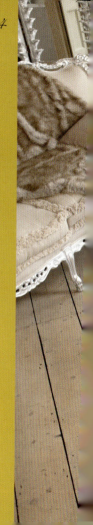

He sits with his legs outstretched and parted. She faces him and lowers herself onto his penis, extending her legs over his so that they point out past his back. His arms encircle her, supporting her upper back, and her hands grasp the outside of his upper arms. Both partners lean back, creating an X-shape with their outstretched legs.

Many women love the sense of surrender and vulnerability this position promotes. With her head flung back to expose her breasts and upper body, and her legs parted to reveal her clitoris and vulva, she can revel in the attention as her lover enjoys the view. Thrusting is almost impossible so it's hard for him to race towards a climax. Clit stim is pretty much impossible without a little outside help, as you're both using your arms to support each other, so invest in a strap-on vibrator that rests lightly on the clit but still gives him access to penetrate. They were made for positions like this. When she comes, the contractions could be enough to make him come without thrusting.

He says: *'I get a second-hand buzz as the vibrations travel through her body and into mine. It's a weird but nice feeling.'*

She says: *'I actually like the act of strapping on the vibe in itself. I like the way it looks on my body and admire myself in the mirror as the straps squeeze into my curves. Just putting it on gets me horny.'*

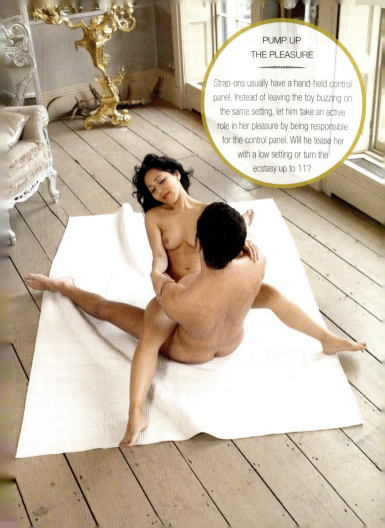

PUMP UP THE PLEASURE

Strap-ons usually have a hand-held control panel. Instead of leaving the toy buzzing on the same setting, let him take an active role in her pleasure by being responsible for the control panel. Will he tease her with a low setting or turn the ecstasy up to 11?

Mild-to-wild rating: 5

THE TANDEM

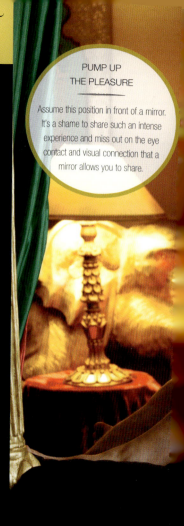

PUMP UP THE PLEASURE

Assume this position in front of a mirror. It's a shame to share such an intense experience and miss out on the eye contact and visual connection that a mirror allows you to share.

Double-headed dildos are usually associated with lesbian sex play, but hetero couples can find plenty of places to accommodate the two-headed beauty.

He sits with his back to her – she places the double dildo on the bed between them, and then lowers herself onto it, penetrating herself vaginally. He then raises his hips and she guides his butt down onto the dildo, using a liberal amount of lube. She controls the pace of the movement and can also reach around to caress her partner's erect penis.

He says: *'I love feeling the scratch of her fingernails down my back in this position.'*

She says: *'I love getting him lubed up, then watching his ass-cheeks part as he accommodates the shaft. It gives me a taste of what it must be like when he uses a toy on me, or puts his dick inside me.'*

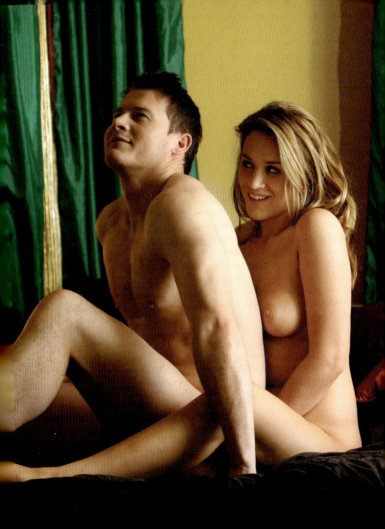

Mild-to-wild rating: 5

Better to Receive Than to Give

Many men crave knowledge of what it must be like to be a woman and to be penetrated. The nearest he'll ever get is experiencing a strap-on dildo – a life-sized penis in a harness that ties around his lover's waist or hips. It can also be hugely empowering for her to experience the thrust and power that penetrating a partner brings.

He bends over the bed or a chair, propping his upper body up on his arms to create the ideal angle for the dildo to enter and sit comfortably in his rectum. She stands behind him, a strap-on dildo firmly attached to her hips, holds his hips, pulls apart his cheeks, applies plenty of lube and slowly enters him, going gently at first, and building up to a pace that he's happy with.

He says: *'The first few seconds are the most intense. I can feel a swell of pleasure as the tip of the strap-on travels over my prostate gland.'*

She says: *'I found a belt that had a little nodule to massage my clitoris. He thought I was pumping in and out extra hard for his benefit but, really the pleasure was all mine.'*

PUMP UP THE PLEASURE

He can give her a 'blow job.' Again, this plays on notions of gender and power. If he kneels before her and takes the dildo between his lips he gets to experience the fullness in his mouth that most women are familiar with. To add to the ecstasy, she can utter commands to him, such as 'Suck my dick.' With his mouth full, he can hardly protest…

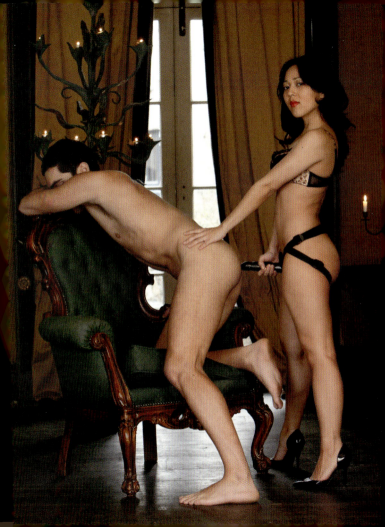

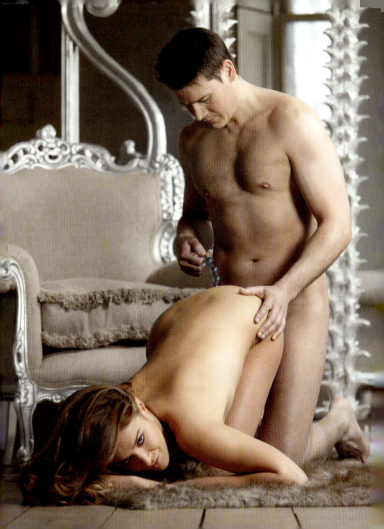

Mild-to-wild rating: 4

BEAD WORK

Love beads are a series of marble-sized beads made of hard plastic strung together on a cord with a loop at one end. They stimulate the prostate gland in men but many women also enjoy the feeling. Because they're small and easy to use, beads are great for people who are new to anal play. If you're having vaginal sex, love beads lend themselves to the doggy position – she kneels on all fours.

First, he inserts the beads one by one into her ass. Then, if she can stand it, he penetrates her vaginally and thrusts, pulling the beads out slowly to send her over the edge. She can return the favour by bending him over and doing the same, although it's important to wash anal toys between partners, even if you're both healthy.

PUMP UP THE PLEASURE

Find out whether fast or slow works best for you – as you approach climax, tease yourself and build up to a rippling orgasm by removing them *slooooowly*. The next time, whip the beads all out at the last minute to trigger an orgasm that could be more intense than any you've had before.

He says: *'Watching the beads disappear into her ass really gets me hot. I'm sure that her pussy feels tighter when she's wearing them, too.'*

She says: *'I love the fact that the anal beads come in these pastel colours. You could mistake them for sweets or a cute plastic necklace but they're not as innocent as they look!'*

Lip service

Oral sex is the most likely way for women to reach orgasm and a treat that men never say no to. Most of us do it in the same old position every time – lying back on the bed while our partner kneels between our legs and licks their lips in anticipation. While that's great, there's a whole world of oral sex positions just waiting to be explored, whether you're giving it, getting it, or doing both at once...

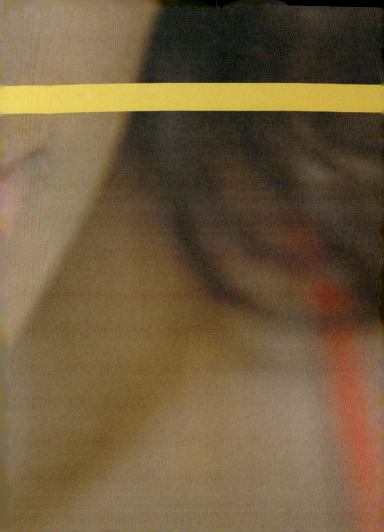

SHE GIVES, HE RECEIVES

TWICE AS NICE

Mild-to-wild rating: 5

This position offers the double delights of her tongue stimulating his anus and perineum (a fine art known as rimming or anulingus) while her hands run up and down the shaft of his penis.

She lies on her back on the bed. He crouches over her so that his anus is hovering just over her face, and gently lowers himself so that his skin is touching, but not crushing her. She raises her knees which he catches hold of to help him balance and breathe. She is then free to reach between or around his legs and slide her hands up and down the shaft of his penis, paying particular attention to the super-sensitive tip, while she explores his ass with her mouth. Alternatively, he can stimulate himself with his own hand while she uses both her hands to part his ass cheeks and delve even deeper. Many men have never allowed their partner to explore the secret pleasure zones of the ass.

> **PUMP UP THE PLEASURE**
>
> If he slips a cock ring over his cock and balls, she can tease him to a longer, stronger erection. When she's had enough, or she thinks he can't take any more, she should easily be able to put him out of his misery... and into the realms of pleasure.

He says: *'I was a bit nervous about having her explore my anus but after some foreplay in the shower I was confident enough to let her boldly go where no girlfriend had gone before. The double sensation of her hands and mouth gave me the strongest orgasm I've ever known.'*

She says: *'It can be a bit suffocating, but if you breathe through your nose you're ok. I was worried about him getting tired and smothering me, but he came so quickly that it needn't have been a concern.'*

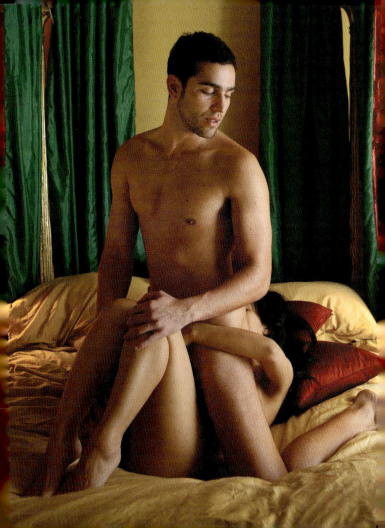

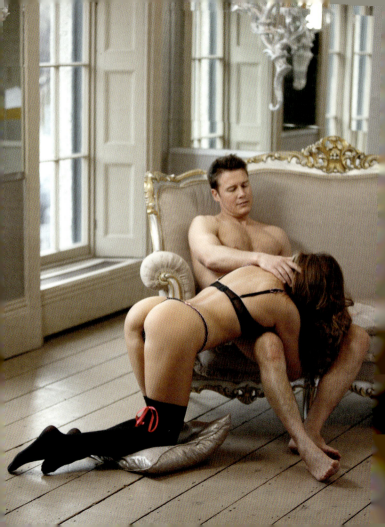

Mild-to-wild rating: 3

Tongue-in-Cheek

She kneels before her man, her body sideways on to his rather than facing him directly. She then takes him into her mouth and, using slow, consistent motions, she gently sucks and licks him to a knee-trembling climax. It's a real novelty for him to find the tip of his penis in the soft hollow of her cheek rather than tickling the roof of her mouth. If he's thrusting too much, she can make her thumb and forefinger into an L-shape until the tiny webbed piece of skin between her thumb and forefinger is taut. By placing her hand at the base of his penis, she can use it as a 'brake' to stop herself biting off more than she can chew.

PUMP UP THE PLEASURE

She decides beforehand whether she wants to swallow and makes the most of her choice. If she's going to do it, she tells him she wants to taste all of him, and licks her lips after the event. If she doesn't, she can still turn his ejaculation into part of the game by asking him to come on her breasts and watch her as she kneels before him and massages his liquid into her skin like a luxurious body lotion.

He says: *'I love the way she looks up into my eyes when she's doing this. It makes me know that even though she seems submissive, she loves what she's doing almost as much as I do.'*

She says: *'I love that moment when his whole body tenses and I know he's going to come. It makes me feel really powerful. I look up at him and think, "I did that."'*

Mild-to-wild rating: 5

TUNNEL OF LOVE

Deep-throating – when he thrusts his penis as far into her mouth as it will go – is a porno trick that most men will have seen but few will have experienced. She doesn't need to be a circus freak sword-swallower but she does need to be in a position where her head and throat are in line, either with her head hanging off the bed or propped up on pillows. This makes a straight line of her throat, and prevents him feeling that his penis has to bend around in her throat. He needs to progress slowly, allowing her to accommodate his dick little by little, and he needs to be sympathetic to the fact that she has to breathe through the gag reflex.

Make the most of the moment when he enters your mouth as, despite its visual appeal, deep-throating doesn't actually feel that great for a guy. When he's in that deep, he'll come into contact with the epiglottis at the entrance to your throat (a soft part of the body that she can't flex or contract), which means that stimulation is minimal.

PUMP UP THE PLEASURE

If this position feels uncomfortable for her – and it can – she can press her breasts together and ask him to finish his thrusting in her cleavage.

He says: *'We tried this but to be honest once my dick was all the way in, I couldn't feel it. It's definitely more about the way it looks and the taboo of the position.'*

She says: *'This was hard work and an unusual feeling. I wouldn't call it unpleasant, but I didn't feel like I could control or pleasure him the way I can if my head is the other way up.'*

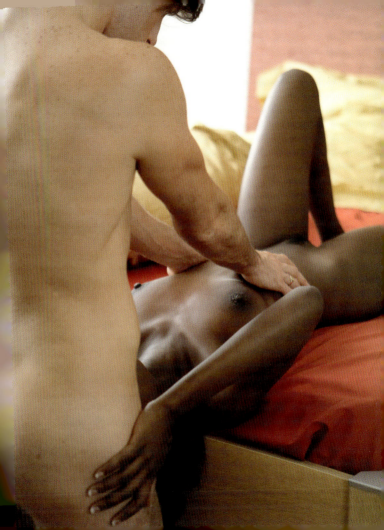

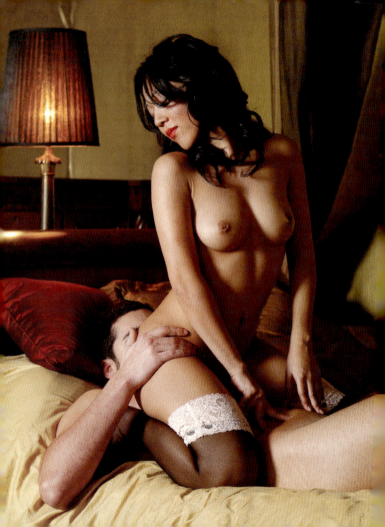

HE GIVES, SHE RECEIVES

QUEEN FOR A DAY

Mild-to-wild rating: 4

A woman sitting on her lover's face is known as 'queening' in fetish circles, and everyone who has tried it either loves or hates it. He slips a pillow under his head and lies still while she gyrates over his lips, tongue and nose (he should never underestimate the pleasure of a well-timed nudge with his nose; to her, in this pose, it feels just like the tip of a penis).

He stimulates her with both upward and downward motions and lots of suction. If she's got her back to him, he's perfectly placed for toying with her anus and perineum. If she's facing him, he'll be in prime position for stimulating her clit. It does require a lot of thigh power on her part not to crush him, which might stop her from relaxing enough to come. If you can't go the distance, use this as a prequel to the classic cunnilingus position, where she lies back and he lies between her legs.

> ### PUMP UP THE PLEASURE
>
> This position is playful as well as intense. She can tease and tantalise her lover by stroking the skin of his chest with a feather tickler while he goes to work on her. If she can make him laugh, the rush of his breath will further stimulate her, and if he wriggles underneath her, she'll feel every twitch of his body.

He says: *'I can tell by the contractions in her pussy when she's about to come, and to tease her, I lay off her clitoris and make my tongue hard and poke it inside her, delaying her orgasm for a few seconds more.'*

She says: *'I had to sink onto all fours when I felt my orgasm coming because otherwise I knew I'd collapse onto his face and suffocate him.'*

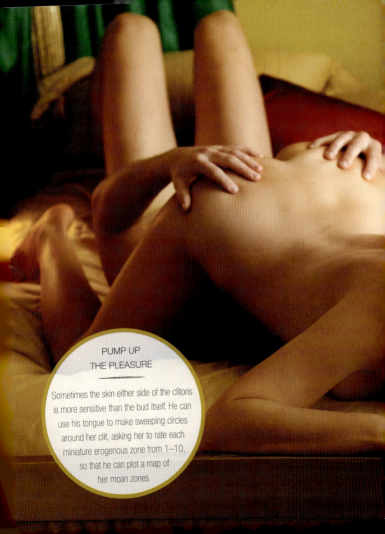

PUMP UP THE PLEASURE

Sometimes the skin either side of the clitoris is more sensitive than the bud itself. He can use his tongue to make sweeping circles around her clit, asking her to rate each miniature erogenous zone from 1–10, so that he can plot a map of her moan zones.

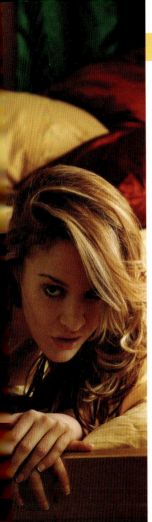

Mild-to-wild rating: 3

Air Kiss

This animalistic pose features her crouching on all fours, with her ass raised into the air like a cat on heat.

He lies on his back on the bed. She crawls over him, making progress up his body, enjoying the skin-to-skin and eye contact, until her hips are level with his face. Then she lowers her head and shoulders down onto the bed, letting her breasts press against the sheets and her ass rise up into the air. Her pussy isn't quite touching his face but they're so close that she can feel his warm breath on her clitoris. He then extends his tongue to caress her clitoris and vulva. She can control the intensity of the stimulation by raising and lowering her ass. If she pulls away from his mouth, she'll experience light, fluttery strokes. If she bears down, the stimulation will be firmer and stronger.

He says: *'I enjoy this most if she has a freshly waxed or shaved pussy because I can access every millimetre of her skin.'*

She says: *'This is a great way to combine oral with full penetration. I can slide back down his body and sit on his dick for a while. It keeps him hard and hungry for more.'*

SIMULTANEOUS STIMULATION

Mild-to-wild rating: 5

ZIG-ZAG

The Zig-Zag looks like position impossible, but actually you're both using your body weight to support each other.

Begin with her crouching over him, with her back to him and her feet on the outer sides of his thighs, while he sits down. Then slowly, she raises her ass up to his face, holding onto his thighs for support, and he leans slowly back. Take each other in your mouths and go nuts.

Although it isn't easy for him to access the clitoris, a strap-on vibe can do some of the hard work on his behalf. You can also happily reverse roles so that he's on top, although you need to be fairly evenly matched in terms of body weight and strength.

PUMP UP THE PLEASURE

This position is all about confidence – confidence that you can support your lover and confidence that you smell and taste good enough to eat. Warming up in the shower together beforehand is a great prelude to passion. Lather each other's genitals using a mild, unfragranced shower gel (soap can strip away her natural juices). Hot water will also help loosen up your muscles before assuming the position.

He says: *'I loved the feeling of bearing her weight – she really sank into my face.'*

She says: *'This was a killer on my thighs and I found that I had to choose between holding the position and relaxing enough to allow myself to orgasm. It's worth it for the novelty value, but I'd never be able to hold that position for the length of time it usually takes me to achieve an orgasm.'*

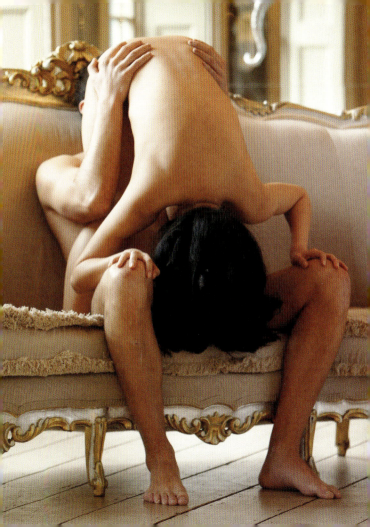

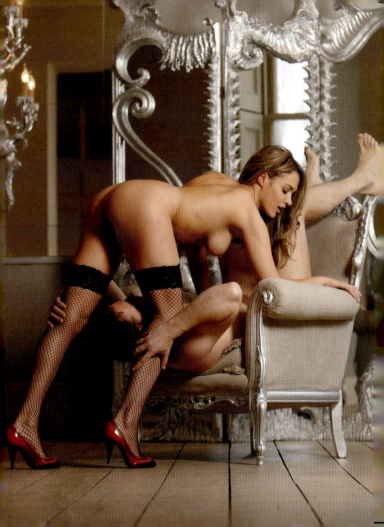

Mild-to-wild rating: 5

THE HONEY POT

He lies back with his head on the edge of the bed or a chair and his legs bent. She spreads her legs and gradually walks over him until her head is bent over his penis and her own genitals are lined up with his face. Both lovers are then in prime position to lick their lips and give great head. She'll probably need both hands to grab onto his hips to stabilise her, but his hands are free to wander to her breasts, clitoris, anus or wherever else she likes to be touched. He can also clasp her waist and give her something to lean on and extra staying power. This position also lends itself brilliantly to coffee tables as they're the right height for her to straddle. Just check it can bear his weight before beginning, and avoid ones made of glass!

> **PUMP UP THE PLEASURE**
>
> You're hungry for each other, so take that one step further. Edible panties, available for men and women, will create a whole new sensation as the soft sugar-paper caresses you, and your lover's tongue and teeth make their way towards the holy grail – your sensitive skin.

He says: *'Usually when she gives a blow job her mouth is the other way up, but in this position you get the tongue on the top of your penis and the roof of her mouth stimulating the underside, which is a real novelty.'*

She says: *'It's not too physically demanding but we found that it's hard to receive pleasure when you're concentrating on what you're doing to your partner. In the end, we took it in turns; I'd stimulate him for a couple of minutes, then he'd kiss me, and that way we both felt the benefits.'*

Faster, harder,

stronger, longer... Ruder

For the following positions, you need to have an open mind and a fit body. They break sexual taboos and physically they can take a while to master, but once you've tried them you've opened the door to a lifetime of potential pleasure.

Mild-to-wild rating: 4

THE HINGE

She lies on her back and folds her legs in so that the fronts of her thighs are pressed against her breasts. He approaches her from the side and gradually bears down on her, pushing her legs further towards her chest. His pelvis is pressed against the backs of her thighs. His arms are out in front of him, supporting him on the bed. When she's as 'folded' as she can go, he gently penetrates her. There is little room for clitoral stimulation in this position. If she's hung up about her butt and doesn't like doggy style, then this is the one for her as the taut positioning of her legs shows her derriere off to its best advantage.

He says: *'The resistance of her leg muscles means that you sort of bounce, rather than thrust, your way to orgasm, which is a delightful novelty.'*

She says: *'This is great if you can't decide whether to have straight or anal sex, and I like to take the time to get him to warm up both areas before I let him know what's on the menu tonight.'*

PUMP UP THE PLEASURE

He can capitalise on the controlling nature of his position by wearing a pair of leather gloves and stroking her skin all over before and during penetration. Black leather is the stuff of sex-with-a-stranger fantasies.

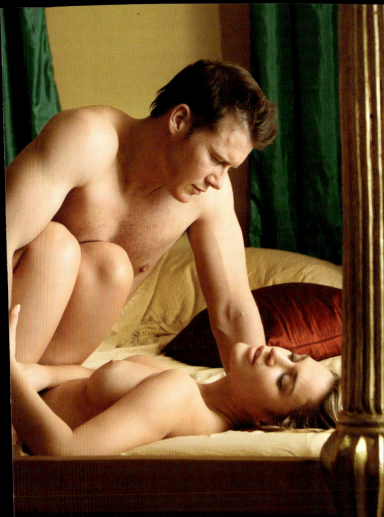

Mild-to-wild rating: 4

THE SIDE SADDLE

Kneeling sideways on the floor, she props one elbow against a bed or a soft chair. She then presses the soles of her feet together, offering him a teasing glimpse of her opening, and slowly raises her upper leg so that he can kneel behind and to the side of her and penetrate her. Hooking his arms around her thighs, he then raises her off the floor so that all her body weight is supported by her elbow and his hold. She feels wonderfully weightless but because this position is precarious, you might be better off slowly rocking and swinging, rather than thrusting, your way to climax.

PUMP UP THE PLEASURE

Strategically placed pillows under his knees and her elbow can take the strain off the joints and allow you to continue in this position for longer.

He says: *'Penetrating her from a sideways angle was a real novelty – her pussy felt slightly different, and the unusual point of view was a turn-on. Even her breasts hung in a slightly different direction.'*

She says: *'This was hard work but worth it – I felt really safe and nurtured knowing that I was depending on him to hold me up.'*

Mild-to-wild rating: 5

THE SEXY SPIDER

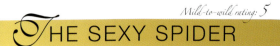

From the side, you'll look like a bizarre eight-legged creature. But you'll be too busy enjoying the unique sensations this position provides to worry about that...

He lies on his back, with only the upper half of his body on the bed and his legs leaning up against a wall. She positions herself so that her back is to him and, using the wall for support, squats onto his erect penis. Penetration needs to be slow until it's firmly established: then, and only then, can he grab her ass and begin to drive himself into her. In this position, his penis rubs against the front of her vaginal wall, stroking her G-spot. Because she's on top, she's in control.

PUMP UP THE PLEASURE

Because this position is so visually compelling, why not try filming yourselves, or set the camera to take some sizzling stills behind you?

He says: *'Just when I was thinking this couldn't get any more intense, she reached between my legs and squeezed my balls gently. I felt my whole body start to quiver but managed to hold the position anyway!'*

She says: *'Penetration here feels really unusual and can take some time to get used to. I could feel his dick tickling my G-spot, but it wasn't possible to do the deep, thrusting strokes I need to come that way. But it was a great precursor to doggy-style sex where I could... and I did.'*

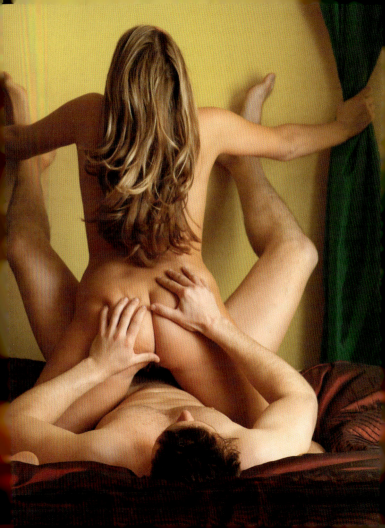

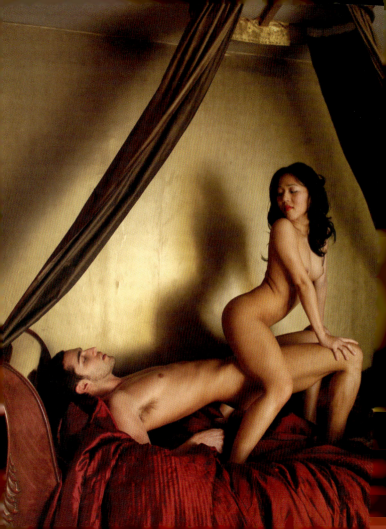

TABLE-TOP MOUNTING

Mild-to-wild rating: 5

There's no better position for him to show off all those hours he's spent working out in the gym than this demanding posture. Make sure you try this one on a bed rather than a hard surface – couples often find that they topple over without warning during Table-top Mounting!

He lies on his back, then props himself up on his elbows, bends his knees and lifts his bottom off the bed so that his torso is almost entirely flat like a table. With her back to him, she slowly sits on his erect penis, keeping her bent legs tight and placing her hands on his knees for extra stability. Like all rear-entry positions, this one has the potential to stimulate her G-spot. It's also great for guys who suffer from premature ejaculation, as the energy needed to maintain the pose diverts blood away form his penis, slowing down his climax.

> **PUMP UP THE PLEASURE**
>
> She might find that wearing a pair of showgirl-style nipple tassels gives her extra confidence to shake and shimmy all over his body. Knowing they're there, but that he can't see them, is a huge tease for him and will only add to the tension in his mind and body.

He says: 'She leant forward and her hair cascaded all over my thighs, tickling and caressing me, which was a nice contrast to the hard physical work of holding the position.'

She says: 'I felt very light and feminine and supported by him, and the penetration was really snug – his dick felt bigger than I've ever felt it before.'

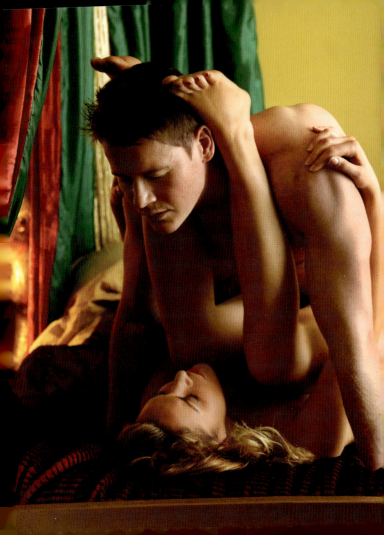

Mild-to-wild rating: 5

Love Lock

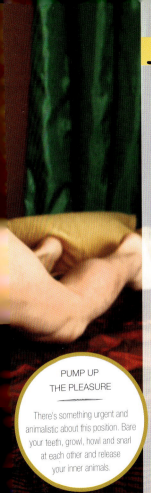

Lying on her back, she pulls her legs together and towards her body. He leans over her, taking his weight on his hands, which are placed near her head, and the balls of his feet. She hooks her ankles around his neck and grabs his arms for added leverage and support. He slides into her in a deliberate, slow, controlled movement.

There's plenty of scope for talking and eye contact, unusual in such an animalistic, carnal position. Plus, his body is pressing against her vulva, a super-erogenous zone that sometimes gets overlooked in favour of its neighbours, the clitoris and vagina.

He says: *'I feel like a caveman as I lean over her, about to ravish her. I love to have sex in this position after I've been chasing her around the house.'*

She says: *'It took a while to get comfortable in this position, but once I worked out that putting a pillow under my hips would change the angle of my pelvis, it was like, wow! It lets you enjoy all of the sensations of that deeper penetration without putting any of the effort in.'*

PUMP UP THE PLEASURE

There's something urgent and animalistic about this position. Bare your teeth, growl, howl and snarl at each other and release your inner animals.

Anal sex

Anal sex isn't just for boy-boy couplings – lots of women say they love the super-snug feeling of back-door loving, and hetero blokes are often pleasantly surprised to discover the world of pleasure that is the prostate gland, a super-sensitive nodule of pure pleasure a couple of centimetres or so up the front of the rectum.

We've used boy-girl couplings here, but the roles can easily be reversed, with the girl wearing a strap-on to penetrate the guy. They also work for same-sex couples – boy-boy sex doesn't need any extra equipment, but girls might like to use strap-ons or dildos to penetrate each other.

No matter what combination of bodies you're dealing with, anal sex requires lube and lots of it, because unlike the vagina, the anus doesn't produce its own natural juices, no matter how aroused you both are. And even if you're both clean as whistles, you should use condoms, as extra bacteria in this area mean the risk of infection is high.

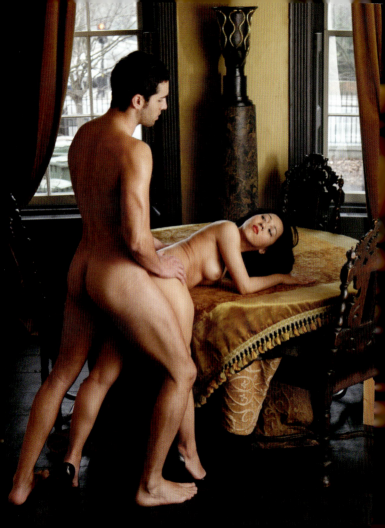

Mild-to-wild rating: 4

BUGGER'S BANQUET

She lies on a bed, or bends over a table or desk, legs slightly bent, while he stands on the floor behind her (or kneels if she's on a bed). He gently parts her buttocks and uses his fingers to lube her up, massaging her anus and checking that she's relaxed, and then he gently penetrates her. His immediate instinct will be to capitalise on the tight penetration by pounding hard, but that might overwhelm his partner. To control his thrusting at first, he can make a ring with his thumb and forefinger and place it just outside the entrance to her anus as a kind of barrier.

PUMP UP THE PLEASURE

If she's already on the dining-room table, why not keep the foodie theme going? Massage flavoured lubes into each other as part of your foreplay, or decorate your bodies with creams and oils that you can't wait to lick off.

He says: 'My balls were slapping against the table with every movement of my hips. This tiny distraction stopped me from coming too soon.'

She says: 'I found that once I was used to the feeling of him inside me, I could alter the position of my legs. For example, if I stretched them out, he felt looser. If I pulled my knees up to my chest, it felt much tighter for both of us – and that's exactly when he came!'

Mild-to-wild rating: 5

DOUBLE DECKER

He lies flat on his back. She squats over him, facing his feet, and slowly lowers her ass onto his erection, tucking her feet in close to his upper thighs. She leans on her hands and bounces up and down, rolling her hips in a gentle figure-of-eight movement to stimulate him. Flexible women can lean back so that their backs are resting on their lover's chest, which will increase the tightness of penetration. Take care when leaning forward in this position as it forces his erection into an unusual and potentially uncomfortable position. Experiment with different levels of leaning back and forth and see how the tightness varies. This position doesn't lend itself to role reversal as men tend to be so much heavier than their partners.

He says: *'If we're not using a toy, I like to slide my fingers in and out of her wet pussy and play with her clitoris in this position.'*

She says: *'As a woman you can feel quite vulnerable during anal sex but actually what I'm doing here is taking the lead. I control the rhythm and depth of the penetration.'*

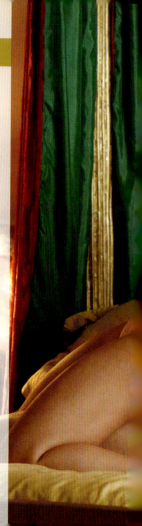

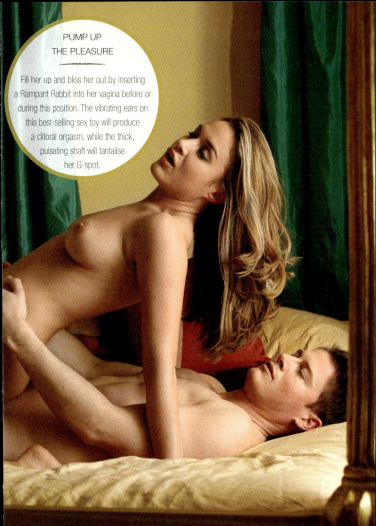

PUMP UP THE PLEASURE

Fill her up and bliss her out by inserting a Rampant Rabbit into her vagina before or during this position. The vibrating ears on this best-selling sex toy will produce a clitoral orgasm, while the thick, pulsating shaft will tantalise her G-spot.

INTO THE DEEP

She lies face down on the bed, making a pillow with her forearms and resting her head on them. Once he slips inside, she slides her legs out as wide as she can. He can remain higher up, supporting himself with extended arms, or he can drop down onto his elbows for extra contact. If he lowers down he should make sure the weight is comfortable for her. Both partners enjoy extra-deep penetration, and because her legs are spread so wide, she gets the added bonus of the bed-sheets creating delicious friction on her exposed clitoris.

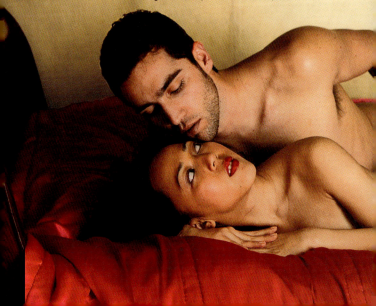

Mild-to-wild rating: 4

He says: *'Seeing her sexy legs spread wide either side of my body was a real turn-on. It felt like an open invitation for me to penetrate her.'*

She says: *'I slid my forefinger and middle finger underneath me and placed them just either side of my clitoris. The pressure of my body weight combined with his meant that I only had to move my fingers slightly to get the extra stimulation I needed to come in this position.'*

PUMP UP THE PLEASURE

Make an already taboo position positively passionate by investing in a pair of leg irons to keep her thighs in the open-wide position.

Lasagna

Mild-to-wild rating: 3

She lies on her front and raises her ass towards him, spreading her legs to make penetration easier for him. He lies on top of her, resting his weight on his elbows, and takes her from behind and thrusts backwards and forwards. This is great for the man who enjoys being in control, because she can hardly move. But this works in her favour, too, as penetration is actually quite shallow and he can't overdo it.

He says: 'What I love about anal sex is the feeling of possessing my partner, and the fact that she was face down on the bed made her surrender complete.'

She says: 'This is a great position if I've already had my orgasm and my clit and pussy are too sensitive to take any more stimulation, but he still wants to come inside me. It's his favourite way to finish off a sex marathon as he knows he's building up to a dirty, deep finale!'

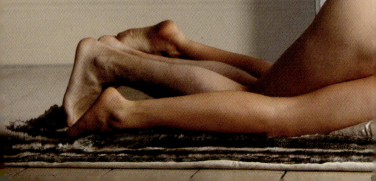

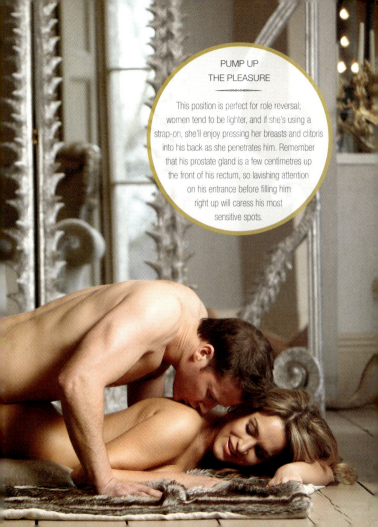

PUMP UP THE PLEASURE

This position is perfect for role reversal; women tend to be lighter, and if she's using a strap-on, she'll enjoy pressing her breasts and clitoris into his back as she penetrates him. Remember that his prostate gland is a few centimetres up the front of his rectum, so lavishing attention on his entrance before filling him right up will caress his most sensitive spots.

I like the way

you move

Now you've tried the hottest and horniest positions in the world, it's time to have a little fun. The following poses all require partners to alter their posture during intercourse so that you never end up quite where you started from. Super-fit bodies aren't necessary to complete these, although a degree of flexibility, a little bit of sexual experience and a sense of humour are all a bonus.

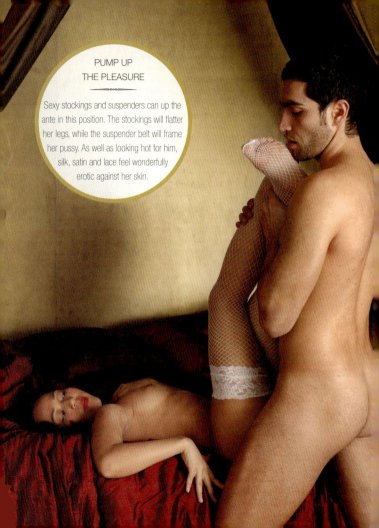

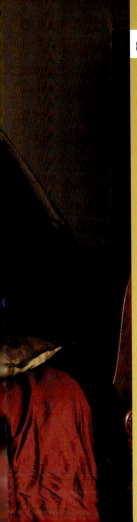

Mild-to-wild rating: 5

NUTCRACKER

She lies on the bed on her back with her ass on the edge and her legs up straight in the air. He kneels at the edge of the bed. After entering her, he grabs her legs, crosses them, and holds them in front of his face. He can cross and uncross them as you make love, so that her legs make a constant, scissoring motion. The sensation of her pussy squeezed tight in tandem with the deep thrusting when she's spread wide open gives both partners lots of variety and allows you to experience lots of sensations without changing position.

He says: *'As I moved her legs in front of me, I felt like I was literally pumping my way to orgasm like she was a giant machine to massage my penis. Plus, the view was amazing.'*

She says: *'Because my pussy was constantly being manipulated – stretched or snug depending on where my legs were – each thrust felt completely different. This made it harder to build up the steady stimulation I need to come, but luckily I had easy access to my clitoris, so I stroked myself while he watched.'*

Mild-to-wild rating: 3

HEADS UP

This is a twist on the missionary position, whereby once he enters her, she pulls her legs together tight, essentially sandwiching his penis and adding delicious friction with each thrusting motion. He then raises and lowers his body above her as though he were doing press-ups in the gym. There is plenty of genital contact, and each time he moves his body up or down, the angle of his penis is altered, stimulating her from the inside out. It's an interesting alternative to the in-out thrust of regular man-on-top sex and one that she might find produces a stronger orgasm in her. The tight, warm grip around his penis when he's in the 'up' position will have him throbbing with ecstasy in record time.

He says: *'This is such a simple twist on the same old man-on-top sex, but I really notice the difference. Penetration is much snugger and tighter and I like to arch my back as I climax.'*

She says: *'I love the feeling of his weight on top of me during missionary, but his head usually ends up buried in my shoulder. Here, I can watch his expression as he comes, which I really get off on.'*

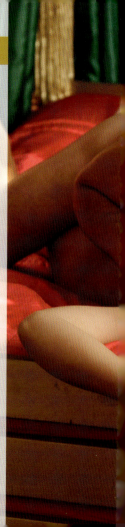

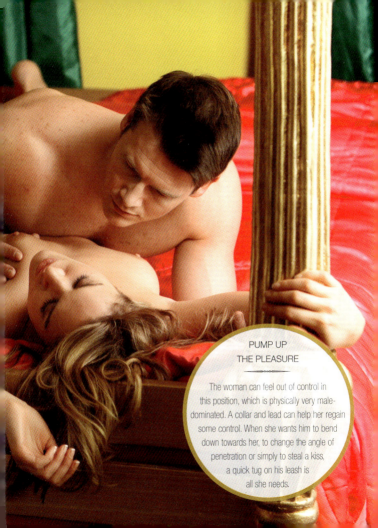

PUMP UP THE PLEASURE

The woman can feel out of control in this position, which is physically very male-dominated. A collar and lead can help her regain some control. When she wants him to bend down towards her, to change the angle of penetration or simply to steal a kiss, a quick tug on his leash is all she needs.

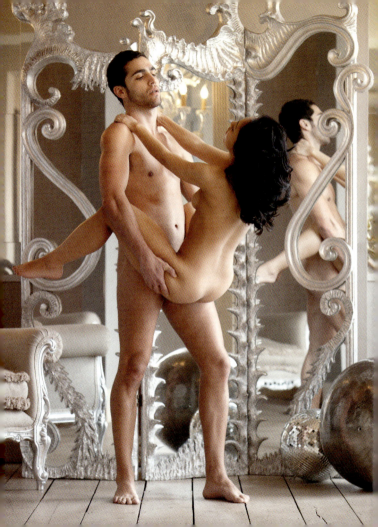

SWING OUT SISTER

Mild-to-wild rating: 4

She wraps her arms around his neck, and with help from him, she wraps her legs around his waist, in the process of lining her vagina up with his penis so that he can enter her. This obviously requires strength and co-ordination on the part of both lovers, so manoeuvring into this position is slow and controlled. Once she's comfortably penetrated, let the swinging begin!

PUMP UP THE PLEASURE

If you really like this, but find it too physically demanding, it could be worth investing in a sex swing to achieve the same sensations but with a percentage of the effort.

He says: *'You'd be surprised to know that the tricky part is not carrying her but lining her up so that penetration is possible. Once that happens, you fall into a natural rhythm very quickly.'*

She says: *'I loved the primal show of strength from my man in this position.'*

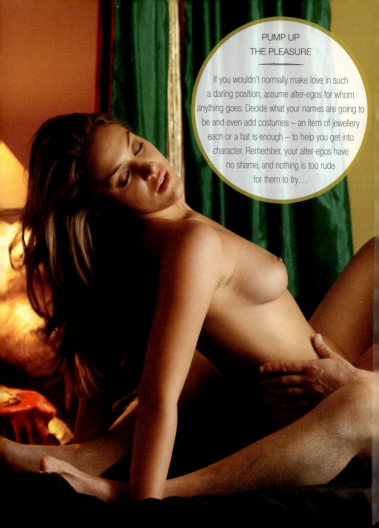

PUMP UP THE PLEASURE

If you wouldn't normally make love in such a daring position, assume alter-egos for whom anything goes. Decide what your names are going to be and even add costumes – an item of jewellery each or a hat is enough – to help you get into character. Remember, your alter-egos have no shame, and nothing is too rude for them to try…

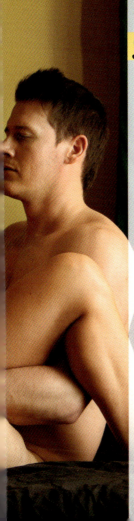

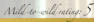
Mild-to-wild rating: 5

Rock My World

Do this one on the bed because you're going to be rocking back and forth and will want lots of padding under those sensitive spines!

He lies back on the pillows while she straddles him, her legs bent and her feet flat on the bed. She slides onto his erect penis. Once they're joined, he should slowly sit upright and bend his knees so that they are pointed slightly outward at a 45-degree angle. His arms come under her knees and rest on her back for support. Hold the position to get used to it for a few moments then rock back and forth!

This position offers shallow penetration, which might not sound great but actually has more passion potential than deep thrusting. The first third of his penis and the first third of her vagina are where most of the sensitive, pleasure-packed nerve endings live, so you're actually stimulating the parts most likely to make you climax.

He says: *'She had to squeeze me with her pussy to hold me in, which I wasn't complaining about.'*

She says: *'I loved reaching in for a kiss mid-way through this. It's really intimate. The rocking sensations are soothing.'*

Mild-to-wild rating: 4

Spinning Jenny

This daring position has the woman rotating on top of her lover.

He lies on his back while she squats down onto his erect penis, her feet near his hips and keeping her legs bent. To warm up and stretch both partners' genitals in advance of this acrobatic act, she gyrates her hips in tiny circles and figure-eights. Then she slowly rotates to the side, using her hands and feet and counting on his support until she's facing his feet. He can stimulate her clitoris or her anus depending on where she's facing at any given point in her spin cycle. Most couples find that after one complete rotation, they're dying for her to lean forward and begin bouncing and thrusting in a classic woman-on-top position.

> **PUMP UP THE PLEASURE**
>
> Slip and slide around by covering yourselves in lube or massage oil and making love on a rubber or plastic sheet.

He says: *'It was a blast to sit back and enjoy this crazy ride. I got to view her from every angle.'*

She says: *'This literally stimulates every tiny part of my vagina. I could feel his dick deep inside places I didn't even know existed. It was great to take it slow and make a note of all the new and exciting feelings I was experiencing.'*

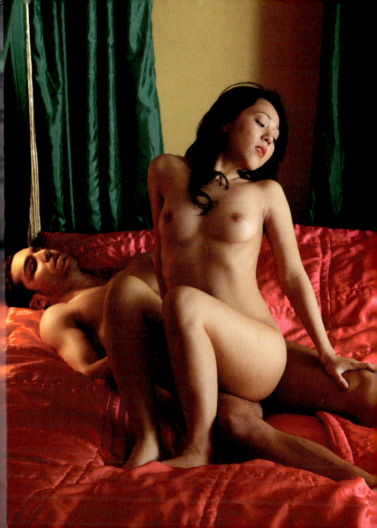

Text Written by Siobhan Kelly copyright © Ebury Press 2010
Photographs copyright © John Freeman 2010

All rights reserved. No part of this publication may be reproduced, stored in a retrieval system, or transmitted in any form or by any means, electronic, mechanical, photocopying, recording or otherwise, without the prior permission of the copyright owner.

Published in the U.S. by
Amorata Press,
An imprint of Ulysses Press
P.O. Box 3440
Berkeley, CA 94703
www.amoratapress.com

First published as *Red Hot & Even Ruder Positions* in Great Britain in 2010 by Ebury Press, Random House

5 7 9 10 8 6

ISBN13: 978-1-56975-729-1
Library of Congress Control Number: 2009905524

Art direction and design by seagulls.net
Photography by John Freeman
Digital systems operator: Erin Eve
Make-up by Chantelle Queenbarrows

Printed and bound in Singapore by Tien Wah Press

Distributed by Publishers Group West